Cumulative Record of Clinical Learning Experience for Post Basic BSc Nursing

CLINICAL LEARNING RECORD LOG BOOK

SN Nanjunde Gowda
MSc (N) DPN PhD
Principal
Anil Baghi College of Nursing
Ferozepur, Punjab, India

Name of the Institution --

Name of the Candidate --

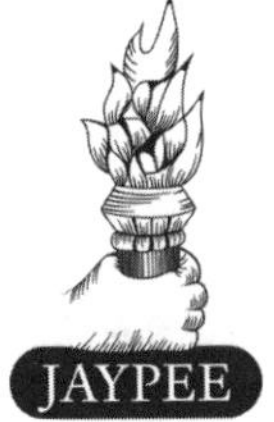

JAYPEE BROTHERS MEDICAL PUBLISHERS
The Health Sciences Publisher
New Delhi | London

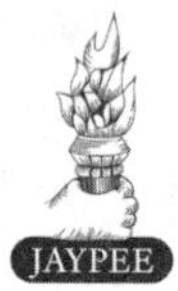

Jaypee Brothers Medical Publishers (P) Ltd

Headquarters
EMCA House, 23/23-B
Ansari Road, Daryaganj
New Delhi 110 002, India
Landline: +91-11-23272143, +91-11-23272703
+91-11-23282021, +91-11-23245672
e-mail: jaypee@jaypeebrothers.com

Corporate Office
4838/24, Ansari Road, Daryaganj
New Delhi 110 002, India
Phone: +91-11-43574357
Fax: +91-11-43574314
e-mail: jaypee@jaypeebrothers.com

Overseas Office
JP Medical Ltd.
83, Victoria Street, London
SW1H 0HW (UK)
Phone: +44-20 3170 8910
e-mail: info@jpmedpub.com

EU GPSR Authorised Representative
Logos Europe, 9 rue Nicolas Poussin
17000, La Rochelle, France
Phone: +33 (0) 6 67 93 73 78
e-mail: contact@logoseurope.eu

Website: www.jaypeebrothers.com
Website: www.jaypeedigital.com

Inquiries for bulk sales may be solicited at: jaypee@jaypeebrothers.com

Cumulative Record of Clinical Learning Experience for Post Basic BSc Nursing

First Edition: 2015

Reprint : 2025, **2026**

ISBN 978-93-5152-349-9

Printed at: Sterling Graphics Pvt. Ltd. India.

Nursing Code of Professional Conduct

Statements/Guidance

1. Act always in such a manner as to promote and safeguard the interests and the well-being of the patients/clients.
2. Ensure that no action or omission on your part or with your sphere of responsibility is detrimental to the interest, condition or safety of patients/clients.
3. Maintain and improve your professional knowledge and competence.
4. Acknowledge any limitation in your knowledge and competence and decline any duties or responsibilities unless you are not able to perform them in a safe and skilled manner.
5. Work in an open and cooperative manner with patients, clients and their families, foster their independence, recognize and respect their involvement in the planning and delivery of care.
6. Work in a collaborative and cooperative manner with health care professional and other involved in providing care, recognize and respect their particular contributions within the care team.
7. Recognize and respect the dignity of each patient and client and respond to their need with care irrespective of their ethnic origin, religious belief, personal attributes and the nature of their health problems or any other factors.
8. Report to an appropriate person, authority, at the earliest. Any conscientious objection may be relevant to your professional practice.
9. Avoid any abuse of your privileged relationship with patients and clients and of the privileged access allowed to their person, property, residency or work place.
10. Protect all confidential information concerning patient's obtained in the course of professional practice and make its disclosure only with the consent or when required by the order of court or where you can justify disclosure in the wider public interest.
11. Report to an appropriate person or authority having regard to the physical, psychological and social effect on cilents. Any circumstances in the environment of care could jeopardize standard of practice.
12. Report to an appropriate person or authority at any circumstances in which safe and appropriate care for the patient cannot be provided.
13. Report to an appropriate person or authority where it appears that the health or safety of the client is at risk, these circumstances may compromise standard of practice and care.
14. Refuse gifts, favor or hospitality from patients currently on your care which might be interpreted as seeking to exert influence to obtain preferential consideration.

The Purpose of the Code of Professional Conduct is to

- Inform the professionals of the standard of professional conduct required of them in the exercise of their professional accountability and practice
- Inform the public, other professionals and employers of the standard of professional conduct that they can expect of a registered practitioner as a registered practitioner.

As a Registered Nurse or Midwife, You Must

- Protect and support the health of individual patients and clients
- Protect and support the health of the wider community
- Act in such a way that justifies the trust and confidence the public have in you
- Uphold and enhance the good reputation of the profession
- Protect self from any harm that might affect own professional performance.

You are personally accountable for your practice. This means that you are answerable for your actions and omissions, regardless of the advice or direction from another professional.

You have a duty of care to your patient and clients, who are entitled to receive safe and competent care.

You must adhere to the law of the country in which you are practicing.

PREFACE

Education technology refers to the development of various methods of educational technological inventions, these advances comes from the interaction of changing concepts with changing techniques leading to new ways of performing educational activities.

Basic of nursing education depending on theory and clinical exposure. The quality of nursing education only gained through theory and clinical experience, nursing educator have the greater responsibilities to develop psychomotor and technical skills with the learner, if the theory and clinical experience systematically planned organized and adhering to the criteria, only we can expect nursing care skills are imparted in the learner the nursing educational institute play a vital role in providing clinical learning experience according to prescribed educational requirement.

The clinical teacher responsibilities to discuss student progress and clinical performance on a continuous basis. Strengths and weakness of the students to be identified and documented and reported the students' signature on each subject only indicates that she/he has been practiced.

This cumulative clinical learning activities record book is designed according to Indian Nursing Council (INC) syllabus and various health university norms for, Post Basic BSc Nursing course.

SN Nanjunde Gowda

Clinical Learning Record

PHOTO
GRAPH

Name of the Institute --

Name of the Student --

Name of the Father --

Date of Birth --

Batch --

Date of Joining --

Date of Course Completion --

Roll Number/Register No. --

Permanent Address --

Signature of the Student --Date--

Name and Signature of Class Coordinator------------------------- Name and Signature of Clinical Instructor -------------------------

Principal Signature

Courses of Study

First Year Hours of Instruction

S. No.	Subject	Theory		Practical	
		Prescribed hours	Allotted hours	Prescribed hours	Allotted hours
1.	Nursing foundation	45		–	
2.	Nutrition and dietetics	30		15	
3.	Biochemistry and biophysics	60		–	
4.	Psychology	60		15	
5.	Microbiology	60		30	
6.	Maternal nursing	60		240	
7.	Child health nursing	60		240	
8.	Medical surgical nursing	40		270	
9.	English	60		–	
	Total	**475**		**810**	

Second Year Hours of Instruction

S. No.	Subject	Theory		Practical	
		Prescribed hours	Allotted hours	Prescribed hours	Allotted hours
1.	Sociology	60		-	
2.	Community health nursing	60		240	
3.	Mental health nursing	60		240	
4.	Introduction to nursing education	60		75	
5.	Introduction to nursing administration	60		180	
6.	Introduction to nursing research and statistics	45		120	
	Total	**345**		**855**	

Post Basic BSc Nursing
First Year Procedures

First Year Post Basic BSc Nursing Procedures

Medical Surgical Nursing

S. No.	Procedures	Demonstration by teacher in laboratory/ hospital		Redemonstration in clinical area by students	
		Date	Signature of teacher	Date	Signature of nursing in-charge/clinical demonstrator
1.	**Comprehensive nursing care**				
a.	History taking				
b.	Physical examination				
c.	Identification of health problem				
d.	Understanding family structure and function				
e	Understanding care giver role				
f.	Review with client daily work schedule				
2.	**Function of Nurse in outpatient department** • Reception of patient • Assessment • Assisting for diagnostic procedures • Assist in admission/referral of patient				
3.	**Nursing in intensive care unit**				
a.	Obtain 12 lead ECG				
b.	Administer oxygen (different method)				
c.	Cardiac monitoring				
d.	Obtain base line specimen for laboratory test				
e.	Analyze pulse oximetry				
f.	Assist in endotracheal intubation				
g.	Perform care in tracheostomy				
h.	Assist in ventilator setting				
i.	Assist in hemodynamic monitoring				
j.	**Maintaining artificial airway** • Maintaining correct tube placement • Maintaining proper cuff inflation • Monitoring oxygenation and ventilation • Maintaining tube patency • Assessing for complication • Providing oral care and maintaining skin integrity				
k.	CVP				
l.	PAWP				
m.	Monitor vital signs				
n.	Monitor level of consciousness				

Contd...

Contd…

S. No.	Procedures	Demonstration by teacher in laboratory/ hospital		Redemonstration in clinical area by students	
		Date	Signature of teacher	Date	Signature of nursing in-charge/clinical demonstrator
o.	Administer emergency medication/blood transfusion				
p.	Monitor response to medication				
q.	Weaning from ventilation				
r.	Prepare for CPR				
s.	Prepare for defibrillation				
t.	Assist in ADL and ambulation				
4.	**Fluid and electrolyte imbalance**				
a.	Assess dehydration				
b.	IV cannulation				
c.	Monitor intake and output				
5.	**Respiratory system**				
a.	Assessment and history taking of respiratory system				
b.	**Assist in diagnostic studies**				
	• Bronchoscopy				
	• Chest X- ray				
	• Lung biopsy				
	• Thoracentesis				
	• Pulmonary function test				
	• Exercise testing				
	• Assist ABGs testing and monitoring				
	• Sputum studies				
	• Blood studies				
	• Radiological studies				
	• Tuberculin skin test				
c.	Assist in inhaler				
d.	Tracheostomy suctioning				
e.	Tracheostomy care				
f.	Assist for intercostals drainage and monitoring and removal				
g.	Assist in postural drainage				
h.	Administer steam inhalation				
i.	Administer nebulization				
j.	Perform chest physiotherapy				
k.	Patient discharge education				
l.	Assist in spirometer				

Contd…

Contd...

S. No.	Procedures	Demonstration by teacher in laboratory/ hospital		Redemonstration in clinical area by students	
		Date	Signature of teacher	Date	Signature of nursing in-charge/clinical demonstrator
6.	**Nursing management of patient with neurological and neurosurgical condition**				
a.	History taking and physical examination of nervous system				
b.	Diagnostic studies assist in /prepare the client for				
	• Lumbar puncture				
	• Radiological examination				
	• Assist in EEG				
	• Electrographic studies				
	• Ultrasounds				
	• Cerebral angiography				
	• Myelography				
	• MRI				
	• CT Scan				
c.	Assist in measuring ICP Monitoring ICP				
d.	Glasgow coma scale				
e.	Preoperative preparation of patient for cranial surgery				
f.	Postoperative management of cranial surgery				
g.	Care of patient with head injury				
h.	Care of patient with skull traction				
i.	Care of the unconsciousness patient				
j.	Care of patient with spinal cord injury				
k.	Drugs used in neurological system				
l.	Patient and family teaching for patient with stroke				
7.	**Nursing management of patient with cardiovascular problems**				
a.	History taking and physical examination of cardiovascular system				
b.	**Blood sample**				
	• FBS				
	• PPBS				
	• GTT				

Contd...

Contd...

S. No.	Procedures	Demonstration by teacher in laboratory/ hospital		Redemonstration in clinical area by students	
		Date	Signature of teacher	Date	Signature of nursing in-charge/clinical demonstrator
	• TFT				
	• CK-MB				
c.	**Blood studies**				
	• CK-MB				
	• Cardiac specific troponins				
	• Myoglobin				
	• C-reactive protein (CRP)				
	• Homocysteine				
	• Serum lipids, cholesterol				
	• Triglycerides				
	• Lipoproteins				
	• Chest X-ray				
	• ECG				
	• Ambulatory ECG Monitoring. Holter monitoring				
	• Exercise treadmill test				
	• Nuclear cardiology Exercise nuclear imaging				
	• Positron emission tomography(PET)				
	• Magnetic resonance imaging(MRI)				
	• Magnetic resonance angiography				
	• Assist in cardiac catheterization				
	• Assist in angiography				
	• Assist in angioplasty				
	• Ambulatory blood pressure monitoring				
	• Serum thyroid stimulating hormone (TSH)				
	• Routine urine analysis				
	• Lipid profile				
d.	Drug administration, monitoring, response to drug, for hypertensive patients				
e.	Drug administration monitoring, response to medication of cardiac patients				
f.	Assist in nutritional therapy (low sodium diet)				
g.	Identification and management of dysrhythmias				

Contd...

Contd...

S. No.	Procedures	Demonstration by teacher in laboratory/ hospital		Redemonstration in clinical area by students	
		Date	Signature of teacher	Date	Signature of nursing in-charge/clinical demonstrator
h.	Monitoring patient with pacemaker				
i.	Assist pericadiocenthesis				
j.	Preparing patient for cardiac surgery				
k.	Postoperative management of cardiac surgery				
8.	**Nursing management of patient with genitourinary problems**				
a.	History taking and physical examination of genitourinary system				
b.	**Assist in diagnostic procedures**				
	• Urine analysis				
	• Urine culture				
	• Urine concentration test				
	• Creatnine clearance				
	• BUN				
c.	**Radiology procedure**				
	• Kidney ureter bladder				
	• Intravenous pylogram (IVP)				
	• Renal ultrasound				
	• CT Scan				
	• Magnetic resonance angiography (MRA)				
	• Cytogram				
	• Uretherogram				
	• Renal scan				
	• Renal biopsy				
	• Endoscopy (cysotscopy)				
	• Cytometrogram				
9.	**Nursing management of patient with gastrointestinal system**				
a.	History taking and physical examination of gastrointestinal system				
b.	Assisting for diagnostic and therapeutic procedure				
c.	Assist gastrostomy feeding				
d.	Insert/monitor/feeding/removal of NGT				
e.	Assist in throat suctioning				
f.	Assist in bowel wash				

Contd...

Contd...

S. No.	Procedures	Demonstration by teacher in laboratory/ hospital		Redemonstration in clinical area by students	
		Date	Signature of teacher	Date	Signature of nursing in-charge/clinical demonstrator
g.	Administering enema				
h.	Assisting in ostomy care				
i.	Assisting in colostomy care				
j.	Prepare and assist patient for: • Barium meal • Barium enema • Proctoscopy • Endoscopy • Liver biopsy • Liver function test • Abdominal paracentesis				
k.	Maintaining intake and output chart				
l.	Preparing patient for general surgery (GI system) • Preoperative preparation participate in: — Physical preparation — Physiological preparation — Psychological preparation — Legal preparation — Preparation day before surgery — Preparation day of surgery — Preoperative check list — Transporting patient to operation room • Intraoperative nursing participate in: — Preparation of operation theater — Packaging of instruments for surgery — Scrubbing, gowning, gloving — Assisting circulating nurse — Assisting scrub nurse — Assisting major surgery (10) — Assisting minor surgery (10) • Postoperative nursing — Preparing postoperative unit — Monitoring postoperative patient — Removal of sutures — Dressing the patient				
m.	Postoperative management of general surgery (GI system)				
10.	**Nursing management of patient with endocrine problems**				
a.	History taking and physical examination of endocrine system				
b.	Assisting for diagnostic and therapeutic procedure in endocrine system				
c.	Assist in routine blood/urine/sputum, investigation				

Contd...

Contd...

S. No.	Procedures	Demonstration by teacher in laboratory/ hospital		Redemonstration in clinical area by students	
		Date	Signature of teacher	Date	Signature of nursing in-charge/clinical demonstrator
11.	**Nursing management of patient with musculoskeletal problems**				
a.	History taking and physical examination of musculoskeletal problem				
b.	Assist in application of plaster cast, its maintenance and removal				
c.	Assist in skeletal traction				
d.	Assist in application of skin traction and care				
e.	Assist in application and removal of prosthesis				
f.	Assist in ROM exercise				
g.	Assist in ADL and ambulation				
h.	Assist in amputation and stump care				
i.	Assist in care of patient with internal external fixation				
j.	Assisting for preparation for bone surgery				
k.	Teach and counsel in crutch maneuver technique				
12.	**Nursing management of patient with disorder of female reproductive tract**				
a.	History taking and physical examination of reproductive tract				
b.	Teach breast self examination				
c.	Teach post-mastectomy exercise				
13.	**Nursing management of patient with oncological disorders**				
a.	History taking and physical examination of neoplasm				
b.	Assist in oncology diagnostic procedures				
c.	Assist in chemotherapy				
d.	Assist in radiation therapy				
e.	Assist in biopsy				
f.	Assist in bone marrow transplantation				
g.	Assist in Pap smear				
14.	**Nursing management of patient with burns and reconstructive surgery**				
a.	Assist burn calculation using rule of nine				
b.	Assist in burns fluid calculation using different formula				
c.	Prepare patient for wound debridement				
d.	Maintain fluid and electrolyte balance for burns patients				
e.	Assist wound dressing using aseptic technique				
f.	Assist in preparing patient for reconstructive surgery				

Contd...

Contd...

S. No.	Procedures	Demonstration by teacher in laboratory/ hospital		Redemonstration in clinical area by students	
		Date	Signature of teacher	Date	Signature of nursing in-charge/clinical demonstrator
15.	**Nursing management of patient with common communicable diseases and STD**				
a.	Review national immunization schedule				
b.	Assist for diagnostic procedure related to communicable disease				
c.	Counseling HIV positive patient				
d.	Follows isolation precaution				
e.	Practice universal precaution • Hand washing • Medical asepsis • Surgical asepsis • Use of masks • Use of gloves • Use of gowns • Disposal of wastes				
16.	**Nursing management of patients with disease of eye, ear, nose, throat and skin**				
a.	Assist for diagnostic procedure related to disease of eye, ear, nose, throat and skin • Assist for procedure of ENT, eye, and skin • Eye examination • Eye irrigation • Preoperative preparation for eye surgery • Eye irrigation • Ear examination • Ear irrigation • Preparation for ear surgery • Nose examination • Nose irrigation • Preparation for nose surgery				
b.	Assist in procedure for ENT, Eye and skin				
17.	**Nursing management of patient with blood disorders**				
a.	Assist in diagnostic procedures related to blood disorders				
b.	Assist for blood transfusion				
c.	Monitor transfusion reaction				
d.	Counsel blood donors				
e.	Assist / follow waste management protocol				
18.	**Nursing in emergency**				
a.	Perform and assist in monitoring and managing crash trolley				
b.	Perform and assist CPR				

Contd...

S. No.	Procedures	Demonstration by teacher in laboratory/ hospital		Redemonstration in clinical area by students	
		Date	Signature of teacher	Date	Signature of nursing in-charge/clinical demonstrator
c.	• Assessment of neurological status • Assist in defibrillator • Assess, perform emergency procedures • Care of patient dying and care of body after death				
19.	**Nutrition and diet**				
	Participate in preparation of food • Liquid diet • Semisolid diet • Solid diet • Low fat diet • High protein diet • Diabetes diet • Salt free diet • Bland diet				

Nursing Care Plan

S. No.	Date	Disease condition	Signature of clinical instructor
1.			
2.			
3.			
4.			

Nursing Case Study

S. No.	Date	Disease condition	Signature of clinical instructor
1.			
2.			
3.			
4.			

Signature of Student

Signature of Clinical Instructor

Signature of Class Coordinator

Signature of Principal

Practical Examination

Medical Surgical Nursing

Signature of Internal Examiner
Date

Signature of External Examiner
Date

Signature of Internal Examiner
Date

Signature of External Examiner
Date

Signature of Internal Examiner
Date

Signature of External Examiner
Date

Signature of Internal Examiner
Date

Signature of External Examiner
Date

Clinical Performance Evaluation

Medical Surgical Nursing

Name of the student -- Level of students --

Hospital------------------ Area ---------------- Date of case study clinical experience started --

Date ended ---------------------------------- Name of the patient ------------------------------ Diagnosis --------------------------------

Name of the clinical teacher in-charge --

S. No.	Criteria	Excellent 4	Good 3	Average 2	Satisfactory 1	Poor 0
1.	**Assessment** Obtain a baseline data and collect history					
2.	Perform a physical examination					
3.	Identifies basic needs of patients, based on assessment and history					
4.	Understanding patient disease condition					
5.	**Diagnosis** Categorizes the patients needs/problems					
6.	Formulates nursing diagnosis as per priority					
7.	**Planning** Plans nursing actions for each needs of the patient					
8.	State the outcome criteria/ objectives					
9.	Involve patient and family members while planning					
10.	Prioritizes the patient needs					
11.	**Implementation** Implements nursing care competently, safely, and accurately within a given time					
12.	Compare laboratory investigation and clinical findings with patients data					
13.	Maintains safe environment for patient and apply scientific principles					
14.	Records and reports patients information accurately					
15.	Follow the principles of drug administration					
16.	Maintains accuracy and economy while giving care					
17.	Gives health instructions to patient and family					
18.	**Evaluation** Identifies out come criteria used to evaluate the patients response to nursing care					
19.	Collects data related to identified criteria					
20.	Re-examine the patient's care plan					

Contd...

S. No.	Criteria	Excellent 4	Good 3	Average 2	Satisfactory 1	Poor 0
21.	Modifies the care plan as per need					
22.	Establishes and maintains outstanding working relationships					
23 .	**Behaviors** punctual for all duties					
24.	Accept constructive comments					
25.	Bibliography					

Total marks

Scored marks:

1–50 marks = poor

51–60 marks =average

61–70 marks = good

> 70 marks = excellent

Signature of Student

Signature of Clinical Supervisor

Signature of Principal

First Year Post Basic BSc Nursing Procedures

Maternal Nursing

S. No.	Procedures	Demonstration by teacher in laboratory/ hospital		Redemonstration in clinical area by students	
		Date	Signature of teacher	Date	Signature of nursing in-charge/clinical demonstrator
	Antenatal care				
1.	Assist in teaching planned parenthood				
2.	Observe different methods of family planning				
3.	Assist in diagnostic procedures of pregnancy				
4.	Antenatal case assessment				
	Intranatal care				
5.	Preparation for delivery				
6.	Assist in teaching pregnant women with HIV and AIDS				
7.	Care of newborn • APGAR score Family welfare • Motivation of planned parenthood • Assist/perform IUCD insertion • Assist/observe tubectomy • Assist/observe vasectomy				
8.	PV examination				
9.	Normal delivery				
10.	Episiotomy and suturing				
	Postnatal care				
11.	Postnatal assessment				
12.	Breast care				
13.	Postnatal health advice				
	Newborn care				
14.	Care of newborn baby				
15.	Assist in care of the newborn including resuscitation				
16.	Assist and teach in feeding				
17.	Observes small and large for date babies				
	Nursing management of abnormal pregnancy				
18.	Assist in teaching pregnant woman with HIV and AIDS				
19.	Care of patient with abortion				
20.	Care of patient with ectopic pregnancy				

Contd...

S. No.	Procedures	Demonstration by teacher in laboratory/ hospital		Redemonstration in clinical area by students	
		Date	Signature of teacher	Date	Signature of nursing in-charge/clinical demonstrator
21.	Care of the patient with pregnancy induced hypertension				
22.	Care of patient with gestational diabetes				
23.	Observe and assist in care of engorged, cracked nipple, breast abscess and mastitis				
24.	Assist and observe obstetrical emergencies				
25.	Assist/observe in forceps/vacuum delivery				
26.	Provide postoperative care for cesarean section				
27.	Drugs in obstetrics Assist in administering drugs during, pregnancy, labor and puerperium on mother and baby				
28.	Observe and assist in counseling infertile couple/ problem associated with unwanted pregnancy/unwed mothers				
	Requirements				
29.	Antenatal examination: 20				
30.	Postnatal examination: 20				
31.	Per vaginal examination: 20				
32.	Conduct normal delivery: 20				
33.	Motivation of planned parenthood: 10				
34.	Stitching of episiotomy				
35.	Witness cesarean section: 10				

Signature of Student

Signature of Clinical Instructor

Signature of Class Coordinator

Signature of Principal

Practical Examination

Maternal Nursing

---	---
Signature of Internal Examiner Date	Signature of External Examiner Date
---	---
Signature of Internal Examiner Date	Signature of External Examiner Date
---	---
Signature of Internal Examiner Date	Signature of External Examiner Date
---	---
Signature of Internal Examiner Date	Signature of External Examiner Date

Maternal Nursing
Clinical Performance Evaluation

S. No.	Activities	5 Excellent	4 Very good	3 Good	2 Average	1 Poor
1.	Take complete obstetrical history, conduct physical examination					
2.	Collect routine lab specimen, transport, labels accurately					
3.	Inspect and palpate the abdomen of antenatal mothers					
4.	Check the fetal heart sound					
5.	Prepare the women for labor					
6.	Keep ready the equipment for normal labor and resuscitation for mother and baby					
7.	Observe and assist normal labor					
8.	Assist in examining placenta					
9.	Give internatal care to mother					
10.	Assist to examine newborn and examine congenital abnormalities					
	Behaviors					
11.	Emotionally well balanced and matured					
12.	Punctual for all duties					
13.	Accepts constructive comments					
	Knowledge					
14.	Demonstrate evidence of self learning					
	Safety					
15.	Provide clean and safe environment to the women					
16.	Recognize the importance of principles and technique for infection control and biomedical waste management					
	Record and report					
17.	Maintain up to date records and reports					
18.	Maintain partogram					
	Communication					
19.	Communicate effectively with patient, family members and health team members					

Level of experience

Total marks ---

1–51 marks = poor

51–60 marks =average

61–70 marks = good

> 70 marks = excellent

Signature of Clinical Instructor-- --------------------------------

Signature of Coordinator --

Signature of Principal

First Year Post Basic BSc Nursing Procedures

Child Health Nursing

S. No.	Procedures	Demonstration by teacher in laboratory/ hospital		Redemonstration in clinical area by students	
		Date	Signature of teacher	Date	Signature of nursing in-charge/clinical demonstrator
1.	Assess normal growth and development				
2.	Identify difference between child and adult				
3.	History taking				
4.	a. Physical examination b. Collection of specimen • Urine • Blood • Throat swab				
5.	Prepare the child for operation (preoperative preparation) • Physiological preparation • Physical preparation • Psychological preparation • Legal preparation				
6.	Assist in administering preoperative medication				
7.	Check checklist before sending patient to theatre				
8.	Assist postoperative nursing care for infant and child				
9.	Assist in pediatrics nursing procedures • Lumbar puncture • Play therapy • Use of restraints • Feeding • Baby bath • Enema				
10.	Assess growth and development from birth to adolescent				
11.	Assist in infant breastfeeding				
12.	Nutritional needs • Participate in anthropometric measurement • Assessment of degree of dehydration • Planning diet for nephrotic syndrome • Protein energy malnutrition • Juvenile diabetes mellitus • Prepare oral rehydration solution				
13.	Nursing care of neonate Assist/participate in • Neonate resuscitation • Phototherapy				

Contd...

Contd...

S. No.	Procedures	Demonstration by teacher in laboratory/ hospital		Redemonstration in clinical area by students	
		Date	Signature of teacher	Date	Signature of nursing in-charge/clinical demonstrator
	• Incubator care • Radiant warmer • Ventilator care • CPR • Exchange transfusion • Follows aseptic precaution				
14.	Participate/assist in history taking and physical examination different system of the child/infant				
15.	Pediatrics emergency assess/assist in • Asphyxia • Convulsion • Head injury • Hemolytic disorder • Burns percentage calculation • Burns fluid calculation				
16.	Participate in calculation of dosage of drugs and administration of medications and injections				
17.	Perform first aid for • Foreign bodies • Hemorrhage				
18.	Enema				
19.	Colostomy irrigation				
20.	Steam and oxygen inhalation				
21.	Visit a center for • Handicapped • Child welfare center • School crèche • Orphanage • PHC/sub center • Indian population project center				

Nursing Care Plan

S. No.	Date	Disease condition	Signature of clinical instructor
1.			
2.			
3.			
4.			

Nursing Case Study

S. No.	Date	Disease condition	Signature of clinical instructor
1.			
2.			
3.			
4.			

Signature of Student

Signature of Clinical Instructor

Signature of Class Coordinator

Signature of Principal

Practical Examination

Child Health Nursing

Signature of Internal Examiner
Date

Signature of External Examiner
Date

Signature of Internal Examiner
Date

Signature of External Examiner
Date

Signature of Internal Examiner
Date

Signature of External Examiner
Date

Signature of Internal Examiner
Date

Signature of External Examiner
Date

Post Basic BSc Nursing

Second Year Procedures

Second Year Post Basic BSc Nursing Procedures

Community Health Nursing

S. No.	Procedures	Demonstration by teacher in laboratory/ hospital		Redemonstration in clinical area by students	
		Date	Signature of teacher	Date	Signature of nursing in-charge/clinical demonstrator
1.	**Assess community health setup**				
2.	Identify the role of personnel working in the community				
3.	Identify epidemiological aspect of nursing				
4.	Participate in community survey				
5.	Assess, plan, implement and evaluate community nursing process based on family needs				
6.	Does family visit				
7.	Assess environmental sanitation				
8.	Participate in immunization program of under five children				
9.	Conduct family health survey				
10.	Participate in national health program				
11.	Assist in counseling family planning				
12.	Assess growth and development of child to adolescent				
13.	Record anthropometric measurement				
14.	Provide care for minor aliments • Fever • Diarrhea • Cough				
15.	Teach care of • Newborn • Infant • Preschool • Adult • Antenatal mother • Postnatal mother • Old age				
16.	Give health education for tuberculosis (home care)				
17.	Assess nutritional status child to adolescent				
18.	Demonstrate bag technique				
19.	Teach preparation of oral rehydration solution				
20.	Teach giving baby bath				
21.	Participate in school health program				

Contd...

Contd…

S. No.	Procedures	Demonstration by teacher in laboratory/ hospital		Redemonstration in clinical area by students	
		Date	Signature of teacher	Date	Signature of nursing in-charge/clinical demonstrator
22.	Test urine for sugar and albumin (if needed)				
23.	Collect vital statistics				
24.	Participate in maternal and child health program				
25.	Participate in health center activities • Antenatal care • Natal care • Postnatal care (provide cord care) • Under five clinic				
26.	Prepare community profile				
27.	Conduct health education • Individual • Group • Teach handwashing at home • Estimation of Hb % • Scabies treatment • Oral rehydration therapy				
28.	Visit activities of subcenter • Water purification center • Sewage disposal plant • Infectious disease hospital				
29.	Conduct health education to (need based) • Individual • Groups				

Nursing Care Plan

S. No.	Date	Disease condition	Signature of clinical instructor
1.			
2.			
3.			
4.			

Nursing Case Study

S. No.	Date	Disease condition	Signature of clinical instructor
1.			
2.			
3.			
4.			

Signature of Student

Signature of Clinical Instructor

Signature of Class Coordinator

Signature of Principal

Practical Examination

Community Health Nursing

---	---
Signature of Internal Examiner	Signature of External Examiner
Date	Date
---	---
Signature of Internal Examiner	Signature of External Examiner
Date	Date
---	---
Signature of Internal Examiner	Signature of External Examiner
Date	Date

Evaluation Tool for Community Health Nursing Experience

Name of the student -- Year of study --

Batch --- Name of community area ---

S. No.	Criteria	Excellent	Very good	Good	Satisfactory	Poor
	Cognative skill					
1.	Follows principles of community health nursing					
2.	Understands the individuals, families, and significant others					
3.	Identifies the demographic characteristics					
4.	Exhibits skills in history taking and physical examination of individuals and families					
5.	Diagnoses the community health needs of the individuals					
	Technical skills					
6.	Demonstrate bag technique during home visit					
7.	Identifies the demographic characteristics and collect data					
8.	Collect vital statistics					
9.	Collect history and exhibits skills in physical examination if needed					
10.	Provides family welfare services					
11.	Refer the individuals or family to appropriate referral center if needed					
	Professional conduct					
12.	Always well groomed and neat, conscious, about professional appearance					
13.	Punctual, never been late					
14.	Courteous and considerate towards others					
15.	Identifies and accepts the beliefs and practices of others including patients family and community					
16.	Listens to individuals, family, community, co-worker and seniors					
17.	Communicate with various national and international agencies					
18.	Encourage active participation of family and community in their own health activities					

Contd...

Contd...

S. No.	Criteria	Excellent	Very good	Good	Satisfactory	Poor
19.	Participate in national health program					
	Health education					
20.	Identifies needs for health education					
21.	Provides health education as per needs of individuals, family and community					
	Records and reports					
22.	Knows to whom the information to be communicated					
23.	Records and reports patients information accurately					
24.	Use appropriate language					
25.	Decides on specific information to be communicated					

Rating Scale

Excellent = Above 70

Good = 61–70

Average = 51–60

Poor = 1–50

Signature of the Students

Signature of the Teacher In-charge

Signature of HOD

Second Year Post Basic BSc Nursing Procedures

Mental Health Nursing

S. No.	Procedures	Demonstration by teacher in laboratory/ hospital		Redemonstration in clinical area by students	
		Date	Signature of teacher	Date	Signature of nursing in-charge/clinical demonstrator
1.	Classification and assessment of mental disorders				
2.	Identify difference between normal and abnormal behaviors				
3.	History taking and assessments methods for mental disorders				
4.	Perform neurological examination				
5.	Perform mental status examination				
6.	Perform process recording				
7.	Admission of psychiatric patients				
8.	Discharge procedures				
9.	**Nursing care of patients with**				
a.	Anxiety neurosis				
b.	Depressive neurosis				
c.	Obsessive compulsive neurosis				
d.	Phobic neurosis				
e.	Somatoforms disorders				
f.	Schizophrenic disorders				
g.	Affective and organic psychosis				
h.	Childhood and adolescent disorders				
i.	Substance use disorders				
j.	Personality disorder				
k.	Psychiatric emergency				
l.	Mental sub-normality				
10.	**Participate in therapeutic modalities**				
a.	Occupational therapies				
b.	Psychotherapy				
c.	Behavior therapy				
d.	Group therapy				
e.	Family therapy				
f.	Pharmacotherapy				
g.	Electroconvulsive therapy				
h.	Recreational therapy				
i.	Play therapy				

Contd...

Contd...

S. No.	Procedures	Demonstration by teacher in laboratory/ hospital		Redemonstration in clinical area by students	
		Date	Signature of teacher	Date	Signature of nursing in-charge/clinical demonstrator
j.	National mental health program				
k.	Community mental health program				
l.	Child guidance clinic				
m.	Deaddiction center				
n.	Mileu therapy				
o.	Counseling • Premarital counseling • Marital counseling • Individual counseling • Family counseling				
p.	Community psychiatry • Conduct case study • Identify person with mental illness • Assist in mental psychiatry				

Nursing Care Plan

S. No.	Date	Disease condition	Signature of clinical instructor
1.			
2.			
3.			
4.			

Nursing Case Study

S. No.	Date	Disease condition	Signature of clinical instructor
1.			
2.			
3.			
4.			

-- Signature of Student

-- Signature of Clinical Instructor

-- Signature of Class Coordinator

-- Signature of Principal

Mental Status Examination

History Taking

Identification data

Name	Age
Sex	Father/spouse
Education	Occupation
Income	Marital status
Religion	IP Number
Diagnosis	
Informant	
History of present psychiatric illness (according to patient)	
History of past psychiatric illness (according to patient relatives)	
Past medical history Family history	
Personal history	

A General Appearance and Behavior Body built --	
Level of grooming	Normal/stability dressed/overdressed /idiosyncratically dressed
Level of cleanliness	Adequate/inadequate/overtly clean
Level of consciousness	Fully conscious and alert/drowsy/stupors/comatose
Mode of entry	Came willingly/persuaded/brought using physical force
Cooperativeness	Normal /more than so/less than so
Eye to eye contact	Maintained /difficult /not maintained
Psychomotor activity	Normal /increased/decreased
Rapport	Spontaneous/difficult/not establish
Gesturing	Grimace /tics/mannerism
Posturing	Normal posture/catatonic posture
Other movement	Stereotype /tremors/extrapyramidal
Other catatonic phenomena	Automatic obedience/ negativism/excessive cooperation/waxy flexibility/ echopraxia/echolalia
Conversion and dissociate sign	
Compulsive acts or rituals	
Hallucinatory behavior	
Speech	
Initiation	Spontaneous/speaks when spoken to/minimal/mute
Reaction time	Normal/delayed/shortened/difficulty
Rate	Normal /slow/rapid
Productivity	Monosyllabic/elaborate replies/pressured
Volume	Normal/increased/decreased
Tone	Normal variation/monotonous

Contd...

Contd...

Relevance	Fully relevance/sometimes off target/irrelevant
Stream	Normal/circumstantial/tangential
Coherence	Fully coherent/loosening of association
Others	Rhyming/echolalia/neologism

Sample of speech (is response to open ended questions)	**Q:** **A:**
Mood	Objective: labile/angry/hopeless/retarded thinking/thought block/muddled or unclear thinking/thinking/flight of ideas

Thought Stream	Normal/formal thought disorder(specify with a sample of speech
Content Ideas/delusions of	Worthlessness/helplessness/guilt/hypochondrial/poverty/nihilistic /death wishs/sucidal/grandiose/reference/control/persecution/bizarre
Thought alienation phenomena	Thought insertion/thought withdrawal/thought broadcasting
Obsess ional/compulsive phenomena	Thoughts/images/ruminations/doubts/impulsive rituals
Perception	
Hallucinations	
Somatic passivity	
Orientation	**Time** Normal/impaired **Place:** Normal/impaired **Person** Normal/impaired
Attention	Normal/impaired
Concentration	Normally sustained/sustained with difficulty/distractible
Memory	Immediate: intact/absent Recent: intact/absent Remote Intact/impaired
Intelligence(performance in studies)	General information
Insight	a. Awareness of abnormal behavior/experience. Yes/no b. Attribution to physical cause. Yes/no c. Recognition of personal responsibility. Yes/no d. Willingness to take treatment. Yes/no
Judgment	a. Personal: Intact/impaired b. Social: Intact/impaired c. Reaction to situation: Intact/impaired

General information whereabouts --

Practical Examination

Mental Health Nursing

-- --

Signature of Internal Examiner
Date

Signature of External Examiner
Date

-- --

Signature of Internal Examiner
Date

Signature of External Examiner
Date

-- --

Signature of Internal Examiner
Date

Signature of External Examiner
Date

-- --

Signature of Internal Examiner
Date

Signature of External Examiner
Date

Second Year Post Basic BSc Nursing Procedures

Introduction to Nursing Education

S. No.	Procedures	Demonstration by teacher in laboratory/ hospital		Redemonstration in clinical area by students	
		Date	Signature of teacher	Date	Signature of nursing in-charge/clinical demonstrator
1.	**Preparation of teaching methods**				
a.	Lecture methods				
b.	Discussion and group discussion				
c.	Demonstration				
d.	Role play				
e.	Pannel discussion				
f.	Symposium				
g.	Seminar				
h.	Field trip				
i.	Workshop				
j.	Exhibition				
k.	Programmed instruction				
l.	Computer assisted learning				
m.	Clinical teaching methods				
n.	Case methods				
o.	Case presentation				
p.	Nursing rounds and report				
q.	Bedside clinic				
r.	Conference individual and group				
2.	**Preparation of educational media and types of audiovisual aids**				
a.	Graphic aids				
b.	Chalk board				
c.	Charts/graphs				
d.	Khadi graphs/bulletin /carton				
e.	Specimen model/puppet				
f.	Slides/films				
g.	Planning school of nursing organization				
3.	**Participate in preparation of**				
a.	Lesson plan				
b.	Unit plan				
c.	Course outline				
d.	Master rotation plan				
e.	Clinical rotation plan				
f.	Evaluation tool				
g.	Participate in practice teaching				
h.	Participate in service education				

Signature of Class Coordinator

Signature of Clinical Instructor **Signature of Principal**

Second Year Post Basic BSc Nursing Procedures

Introduction to Nursing Service Administration

S. No.	Procedures	Demonstration by teacher in laboratory/ hospital		Redemonstration in clinical area by students	
		Date	Signature of teacher	Date	Signature of nursing in-charge/clinical demonstrator
1.	Preparation of hospital organization chart				
2.	Preparation of nursing unit layout				
3.	Preparation of duty roster for nursing staff				
4.	Maintenance of patients records				
5.	Participate in preparation of job description for nursing personnel				
6.	Participate in nursing staff leave planning				
7.	Participate in performance appraisal				
8.	Participate disciplinary proceeding				
9.	Participate staff development, orientation program				
10.	Participate in inventory taking				
11.	Participate in taking care of equipments				
12.	Participate in reporting				
13.	Budget planning				
14.	Participate in public relation				
15.	Participate in drug indenting				
16.	Participate in preparation of hospital census				
17.	Observe the functioning of various nursing, medical administration				

Signature of Class Coordinator
Signature of Clinical Instructor

Signature of Principal

Second Year Post Basic BSc Nursing Procedures

Research Project

Students will conduct research project in small groups in selected areas of nursing and submit a report (group studies may include studying for existing health practicies. Improved practices of nursing (procedures), health records, patient records and survey of nursing literature.

Project work for small groups

Title of the topic (project topic)

Name of the guide --

Name of the institute --

Name of the students and signature --

Outline for Research Report

What to include in a research proposal

Preliminary section

1. Title page
   a. Approval sheet from head of the institution with college stamp
   b. Approval sheet from research guide and experts with college logo emblem
   c. Acknowledgement
   d. Table of content
   e. List of tables
   f. List of figures
   g. List of appendices
   h. Abstract
2. Introduction
3. Need for the study
4. Title or statement of the problem: A brief description of the proposed study, ideas to include in a title could be:
   a. Nature of the research, for example, a survey or a randomized controlled trial
      - The subject of the research –for example preoperative teaching, wound care
      - The type of subject the research is concerned with, for example patient with breast cancer, patient with diabetes.
   b. Aims and objectives: The specific, concrete and achievable objectives of the research study, often expressed in the forms of question
   c. Operational definitions
   d. Hypothesis (null hypothesis, research hypothesis)
   e. Assumptions
   f. Conceptual framework

5. Justification or rationale for the study: The problem which is being tackled by the research study and why it is important, including description or estimates of the size of the problem and its cost or consequences, it should also explain how the study will add to any previous research on the subject, how it relates to relevant theory, and what the practical implications are likely to be.
6. Literature review: A summary and explanation of the key studies relevant to the proposed project. The review should state clearly how the previous research. This is an opportunity to explain both the theoretical and practical implications of the study.
7. Plan of investigation (method or procedure)/methodology: An outline of the process by which the research will be done. (The plan should include research design setting of the study, population and sample, sample size, sampling technique, sampling selection criteria, inclusion and exclusion criteria, development, description and administration of tool, scoring procedure, medium of instruction, content validity and reliability of the tool, pilot study, the method and / or design, procedure for data collection, attrition of the sample, statistical analysis used for the study).
8. Population and sample: The characteristics of the people who will be the subjects of the study, how a sample of the sample will be drawn and criteria for selecting the sample. The reason for using a particular sampling strategy and the size of the sample should be explained.

   Pilot study: A summary of any pilot study which has already been performed or the plan for the pilot study to be done before the main study is carried out.

   Data collection: The precise measures that will be made and the exact procedure to be followed, including definitions to be used for data collection purposes, the methods that will be used to analyze the data, including any statistical tests, should be described.
9. Work plan: Detailed plan of how the work required for the study will be carried out and the time scale for all the phase of the work.
10. Ethical consideration: A description of any ethical issues in the research study and proposed procedures for handling the issues, including written consents, voluntary participation, and so on.
11. Expected end points and how they will be disseminated: One end product of a research study is a report, but there may be others, such as new research tools or teaching or clinical aids, which should be mentioned.
12. Data analysis and interpretation
13. Discussion
14. Summary of the study findings
15. Conclusion
16. Implication
17. Strength of the study
18. Limitation of the study
19. Bibliography
20. Appendices
    a. Letter seeking permission to conduct the study
    b. Tools/instruments used in the study
    c. Certificates for content validity
    d. Any other modules with validation report
    e. Editors certificate

APPENDIX

Medical Surgical Nursing Clinical Assessment Format

Teacher Instructions for Use of Clinical Assessment Form

Description of the form

There are four major areas of student performance being measured with this form, nursing knowledge, medical knowledge, case studies, and professional conduct. Each area identifies certain standards which must be met in order for the student to achieve the highest marks for that standard is the optimum behavior expected of the student.

Administration of the form

1. This clinical assessment form is to be explained to the student at the beginning of the clinical experience in which it will be used.
2. The clinical assessment form is to be completed by the clinical teacher at the end of clinical posting.
3. At the end of clinical experience, the completed form is to be discussed with the student and an explanation provided for any marks that are not understood by the student.
4. The student's signatures on the form only indicate that the she/he has been presented with the form. if the student disagrees with the marking, the student should write a comment on the form to that effect and may pursue the matter with the coordinator, if their is one or with the principal.

Use of the form

1. Each standard has a four point rating scale with the following definitions:

   a. Standard met: The student achieved all of the items identified in the standard.

   b. Standard almost met: The student achieved more than half of the items identified in the standard.

   c. Standard far from met: The student achieved less than half of the item identified in the standard.

   d. Standard not met: The student did not achieve the items identified in the standard.
2. Each standard has different marks depending on the importance of that standard to the overall assessment. The number of marks to be awarded for each point of the rating scale is listed in under that point.

Medical Surgical Nursing

Guidelines for Clinical Performance Evaluation

Student's name -- Medical surgical unit --
Student's number-------------------------------Ward--------------------------------From---------------------------------To------------------------

Performance Level

S. No.	Standard	SM (4 M)	SAM (3M)	SFFM (2M)	SNM (1M)	SNM
1.	**Nursing knowledge** Assessment and nursing diagnosis					
a.	Collect thorough knowledge about patient illness					Unable to collect data about patient or has no knowledge about patient
b.	Recognizes the physical needs of the patient					Unable to assess patient physically. Needs constant guidance
c.	Identifies psychological needs of the patient and family					Unable to identifies psychological needs of the patient and family
d.	Categorizes the patient problems					Unable to formulate complete nursing diagnosis
e.	Formulates complete nursing diagnosis					Unable to formulate complete diagnosis
2.	**Planning**					
a.	Prioritizes the patient needs					Unable to identify the prioritize needs
b.	Establishes suitable nursing actions for each patient's needs					Unable to plan nursing actions for patient or unable to cope with routine work
c.	Able to organize nursing actions within the given time					Need more guidance and time to plan the nursing care
3.	**Implementation**					
a.	Competent in implementing nursing care thorough, safe and accurate, collects and replaces equipment, organizes activities within time					Demonstrate minimal competence in implementing nursing care. Disorganized, wastes time and energy. Rarely completes work within time
b.	Maintains comfortable environment for patient. Applies scientific principles					Ignores body alignment. Doesn't pay attention to patient discomfort. Ignores scientific principles when carrying out care
c.	Maintains safe therapeutic environment					Unable to maintain healthy, safe and clean environment
d.	Accurately records and reports patient information					Fails to report or record accurate information

Contd...

Contd...

S. No.	Standard	SM (4 M)	SAM (3M)	SFFM (2M)	SNM (1M)	SNM
e.	Able to give planned health instructions to patient and family					Unable to give even incidental teaching to patient and family
4.	**Evaluation**					
a.	Establishes outcome criteria for the patient including physical state, behavior and response					Unable to set the outcome criteria or unable to monitor patient's progress
b.	Able to state rationale for nursing actions					Unable to state rationale for nursing action
5.	**Medical knowledge**					
a.	**Drug file:** Presents written document as follows: name of the drug, action, indications, dosage, ranges, contraindications, side effects, precautions					No written documentation of drugs administered
b.	**Medical diagnosis:** States accurate medical diagnosis) of each patient cared for and describes etiology, signs and symptoms, medical therapy and results of medical therapy					Unable to state medical diagnosis(es) of each patient cared for nor describe etiology, signs and symptoms, medical therapy and result s of therapy
c.	**Laboratory investigation:** States proper names of laboratory investigations of each patient cared for and describe reasons for tests, patient preparation for tests, test procedure					Unable to state name of laboratory investigations of each patient cared for not describe reasons for tests, patient preparation or test procedure
d.	**Case study:** Accurately completes all sections of written case study format and submits on time					Does not present accurate written case study on time
6.	**Professional conduct**					
a.	**Uniform:** Always well groomed and neat, conscious about professional appearance					Pays no attention to grooming and is untidy
b.	**Punctuality:** Exceptionally punctual for clinical and has never been late, completes all learning assignments on time					Consistently late for clinical. Makes no attempt to complete the given learning assignments on time, stops in mid task when clinical hours are over
c.	**Sense of responsibility:** Readily accepts responsibility, reliable, adaptable and displays consistency in work, judgement is consistently sound and logical, works effectively under pressure					Reluctant to take responsibility and avoids it. Likely to make illogical, hasty decisions and tends to lose control under excessive pressure
d.	**Initiative for self learning:** Eager to learn and seek new learning experiences self directives in expanding knowledge and utilizing available resources and has original ideas					Fails to participate in new learning experiences or utilizing available resources to expand knowledge even when directed to do so. Lacks capacity for independent actions and always needs specific directions

Contd...

Contd…

S. No.	Standard	SM (4 M)	SAM (3M)	SFFM (2M)	SNM (1M)	SNM
7.	**Communication skill**					
a.	**Patient and family:** Establishes and maintains outstanding working relationships with patients and families					Fails to establish effective working relationship with patients and families
b.	**Hospital staff/health team:** Establishes harmonious relationship with the members of the health team, deals with them skillfully, smoothly and with insight. Polite and helpful **Colleagues:** Very well accepected by colleagues. Always concerned about them and works well with them					Has difficulty in getting along with other members of the health team and is argumentative Not accepted by the colleague's. Tends to remain alone. Demonstrate little interest in others
c.	**Teachers:** Always respects rules and regulations, accepts constructive criticism					Shows no respect for teachers. Breaks rules and regulations and resents constructive criticisms

Sub total of marks--

Total possible marks --Total marks obtained--

Signature of student--

Signature of teacher --

Date signed --

Key

SM = standard met
SAM = standard almost met
SFFM = standard for from met
SNM = standard not met

Clinical Assessment Tool for Pediatrics Nursing (Child Health Nursing)

Student's name --Hospital--
Student's roll number--Ward--
Instructor's name --
Posting from--To --

Required clinical behaviors	Performance level = comments

S. No.	Required clinical behaviors	SM 3	SAM 2	AFFM 1	SNM 0	SNM = Comments
1.	**Nursing knowledge** **Assessment and nursing diagnosis**					
a.	Collects the data about the child's needs (physical and psychological) during illness					Unable to collect the data about the child's needs (physical and psychological) during illness
b.	Assesses the child's growth and developmental needs					Unable to assess the child's growth and developmental needs
c.	Recognizes the psychosocial development stages					Recognizes the psychosocial development stages
d.	Assesses the nutritional needs of the child					Unable to assess the nutritional needs of the child
e.	Recognizes play needs of the child					Unable to recognize play needs of the child
f.	Assesses the child's parents and family members knowledge about the child condition					Unable to assess the child's parents and family members knowledge about the child condition
g.	Categorizes the child needs					Unable to categorize the child's needs
h.	Formulates nursing diagnoses					Unable to formulate nursing diagnoses
2.	**Planning**					
a.	Prioritize the child's needs according to the developmental stages of the child					Unable to identify the priority the child's needs according to the developmental stages of the child
b.	Establishes and recognizes for suitable nursing actions each child needs					Unable to establish and recognize for suitable nursing actions each child needs
c.	Considers psychosocial needs of the child when planning nursing care					Unable to consider psychosocial needs of the child when planning nursing care
d.	Develops nutritional plan for the child					Unable to develop nutritional plan for the child
e.	Plan play needs					Unable to plan play needs
f.	Involves child, parents and family members in planning for health teaching					Unable to involve child, parents and family members in planning for health teaching

Contd...

Contd...

S. No.	Required clinical behaviors	SM 3	SAM 2	AFFM 1	SNM 0	SNM = Comments
3.	**Implementation**					
a.	Maintains safe and therapeutic environment according to developmental stage					Unable to maintain safe and therapeutic environment according to developmental stage
b.	Thorough safe and accurate in implementing planned nursing care according to the child's needs					Unable to implement. Thorough safe and accurate in implementing planned nursing care according to the child's needs
c.	Meets nutritional needs of the child as planned					Meets nutritional needs of the child as planned
d.	Meets play needs of the child					Unable to meet play needs of the child
e.	Gives planned health education to the child's parents and family members					Unable to give planned health education to the child's parents and family members
f.	Maintain accuracy and economy while giving care					Unable to maintain accuracy and economy while giving care
g.	Accurate in recording and reporting child's significant information to the appropriate personnel					Fails to report accurate and significant information to the appropriate personnel
4.	**Evaluation**					
a.	Evaluates with guidance the care given					Unable to evaluate the care even with guidance
b.	Modifies the plan					Unable to modifs the plan
5.	**Medical knowledge**					
a.	Medical diagnosis: Knows medical diagnosis of each child cared for and able to describe pathophysiology, predisposing factors, etiology, signs and symptoms, therapeutic management and results					No knowledge about medical diagnosis of child cared for and unable to describe pathophysiology, predisposing factors, etiology, signs and symptoms, therapeutic management and results
b.	**Investigations:** Describe investigations done and knows the reasons, preparation and procedures and interprets the result of the specific tests done for the child cared					Unable to describe investigations done and does not know the reasons and interprets the result of the various tests done for the child cared
c.	Medications: Able to describe and calculate the drugs administered, knows the name, action, indications, dosage, toxic effect, precautions and presents written document, for the drugs administration					Unable to calculate the drug dosage did not present written. The documentation of any drug administers to the child care
6.	**Professional conduct**					
a.	**Uniform:** Always well groomed and neat, conscious about professional appearance					Pay no attention to grooming and is untidy
b.	**Punctuality:** Exceptionally punctual for clinical and has never been late, completes all given learning assignments on time					Consistently late for clinical. Makes no attempt to complete the given learning assignments on time. Stops in mid task when clinical hours over

Contd...

Contd…

S. No.	Required clinical behaviors	SM 3	SAM 2	AFFM 1	SNM 0	SNM = Comments
c.	**Sense of responsibility:** Readily accepts responsibilities, reliable, adaptable and displays consistently in work, judgments is consistently sound and logical works effectively under pressure					Reluctant to take responsibility and avoids it, make illogical and avoids it. Hasty decisions and lends to lose control under excessive pressure
d.	**Initiate for self learning:** Eager to learn and seek new learning experiences, self directive in expanding knowledge and utilizing available resources and has original ideas					Fails to participate in new learning experience or in utilizing available resources to expand knowledge. Even when directed to do so. Lacks capacity for in dependent action and always needs specific directions
e.	**Communication skills:** **Children and parents and families**: Establishes and maintains outstanding working relationships with children and family members					Fails to establish effective working relationship with children and family members
	Hospital staff and health team: Establishes a harmonious relationship with the members of health team, deals with them skillfully, and with insight, polite and helpful					Has difficulty in getting along with other members of the health team and argumentative
	Colleagues: Very well accepted by colleagues. Always concerned about them and works well with them **Teachers:** Always respects rules and regulations. Accepts constructive criticism	4	4	2		Not accepted by the colleagues, tends to remain alone. Demonstrate little interest in others. Shows no respect for teachers, breaks rules and regulations as result does not accept constructive criticism

Total marks = 100	**Marks obtained =**
Comments: Student's Signature: Instructor's Signature: Date Signed:	

Nursing Care Plan Format

History Taking and Physical Examination

Nursing assessment frequency and extent of the nursing assessment of any system function are based on several factors, including the severity of the patient's symptoms and presence of risk factors, the purpose of assessment.

The physical examination is used to determine the strengths of the patient or the responses the patient exhibits:

Nursing History

Name of the nursing institute --

Student's name --

Specialty posting --Period from-------------------------------------To--------------------------------------

Demographic Data

Name of the patient	**IP no.**
Age	**Gender**
Marital status	**Nationality**
Language spoken	**Religion**
Occupation	**Home town /city**
Education	**Income**
Date of admission	**Treatment received on arrival to hospital**
Provisional diagnosis	**Name of the doctor who is treating the patient ------------------ and unit ---------------------------**

History of Present Illness

Ask any or all of the following as appropriate and write a summary

Date of admission --

Reason for visit --

When did the symptoms started--

General state of health --

Was the onset sudden or gradual --

How often the problem occurs --

Has the problem occurred before --

Summary --

Treatment received on arrival to hospital --

Chief Complaint

Eliciting a client's history not only assist with individualizing the plan of care but also helps to establish a bond with that client.

Gather specific information regarding onset, location, duration, characteristics, associated manifestation, aggravating and relieving factors.

As a medical surgical nursing nurse standing at the client bedside you may be the first one to see the client and obtain the history

Onset --

Location --

Duration --

Aggravating factors--

Relieving factors --

Associated manifestation --

Past surgical history--

Past medical history --

Allergies --

Medication History

Medication prescribed. Use of anti-hypertensive/ diuretics/vasodilator.

Nitroglycerin/anticoagulant/digoxin/bronchodilators/contraceptive/hormones/steroids/antidepressant/ psychotropic/thyroid hormones/over the counter medication/herbs.

Note time and dosage and how often they are taking.

Allergies

Note and describe any environmental, food or drug allergies.

Relevant Family History

Type of family: Nuclear /joint family

Members of the family: Parents / brothers/sisters --

Family history of illness
Is there any family history of: Asthma/cancer/diabetes/epilepsy/hypertension/heart disease/hepatitis/hemophilia/stroke/ tuberculosis/mental disorders/thyroid or autoimmune disorders aged grand parent and siblings alive? If so what is there current state of health if not state the cause of death and age of death

Any major illness in the family: Yes/ No. If yes specify--

Who is suffering --

What disease --

What is their condition now --

Past health history
Previous hospitalization:
Surgery if any:
History of communicable disease:
Is the client taking any prescription or over the counter medications on a regular basis/ notice all the medications, how long:

Psychosocial and spiritual data
Social support system: Client occupational history. How does illness effect work/study and financial status of the client?

Emotional responses
How does the client appear happy/sad/anxious/irritable?
Body language congruent with what the client saying?
Is the client dressed appropriately/clean/unkempt?
How does the client feel?
What does the client normally do to cope with disease condition?

Cognitive responses
Does the client have an adequate knowledge of his/her illness and treatment?

Health behaviors
Use of alcohol/tobacco. Does the client comply with therapy/drug abuse?
Does the client comply with therapy?

Values and beliefs
What are the clients attitudes/beliefs about hospitalization?
Does he/she have any inappropriate perception of illness?

Dietary Habits

Assess excess or deficit caloric intake and clients approximate intake of foods, high in sodium, cholesterol, saturated fat, and caffeine.

Physical Examination

Use questioning, observation and examination to gather data. Tick items that apply to the client and comment as needed.

Sensation

Eyes

Poor vision -
Eye pain -
Blurred vision-
Itching -
Eye infection—blindness R/L
Prosthesis—glasses/contact lens

Ears

Ringing in ears-
Ear pain-
Discharge -
Itching
Ear infection—loss of hearing R/L
Hearing aids

Tongue

Difficulty of taste

Nose

Frequent colds-
Nose bleeds -
Pain—discharge

Touch

Reduced or tactile perception

Comments

Skin and Mucous Membranes

Skin

Excessive dryness - Bruising - Jaundice Itching
Rash - broken skin/wound - Pale/flushed - Poor turgor
Change in pigmentation

Mouth and Throat

Sore throat - Coated tongue- Dental caries -
Bad breath (halitosis) - Bleeding gums - Dentures upper/lower

Hair

Itchy scalp - Hygiene poor - Dandruff - Hair change
Loss/excess

Nails

Colors changes - Biting - Spliting - Clubbing

Comments

Respiration

Rate ----------------
Characteristics ---------------------------------------

Cough - Dyspnea - Wheezing - Coughs blood (hemoptysis)
Cyanosis - Pain on breathing - Restlessness - Smoke (how many per day)

Comments

Circulation

Pulse rate ------------------------------/Min characteristics ------------------------------
Blood pressure --mm Hg
Fatigue - Chest pain - Nausea - Vomiting –
Anemia - varicose veins - Peripheral pulses - Leg swelling/ulcers

Comments

Nutrition

Weight -- Height --Skin fold thickness --------------------------

Appetite change - Weight change - Nausea Vomiting -----

Dysphasia- Heart burn - Dentures—upper/lower

Normal eating pattern (likes and dislikes

Comments

Abdomen

Inspection: Rasheses- Lesions Scar/ striae Distended

Perstalsis.present/absent Tenderness/ mass

Elimination

Urinary

Frequency - Urgency - Dribbling - Urinary incontinence

Painful urination Retention Dysuria Urinary appliance

Nocturia Hematuria Anuria Distended bladder

Activity /Exercise

Muscle pain Muscle weakness Cramps Joint pain/swelling

Stiffness of movements Deformities Abnormal gait Fatigue

Impaired coordination

Self care (describe limitation to eating, bathing, dressing, toileting, ambulating)

Comments

Comfort

Describes the following

Pain if yes how it is relieved

Sleep pattern and methods/treatment used for sleep

Neurological Responses

Disorientation Unconscious Headache Tremors
Paralysis Numbness Weakness Seizures (fits)
Dizziness Loss of memory Difficult expressing self verbally

Comments

Immune Response

Temperature --

Allergies - Fever in last 45 hours - Swollen glands

Chemotherapy--

Comments --

Sexuality

Female

Age of menarche ------------------------------LMP ------------------------------Duration ----------------------

Flow ------------------------------Cycle ------------------------------ (days)

Dysmenorrheal - Bleeding between periods Vaginal bleeding

Males

Discharge - Swelling/masses

Comments --

Investigation Done

Date	Name of the investigation	Normal values	Patients values/result	Significance

Medical diagnosis (final) --

Drug Management

Name of the drug	Dosage and frequency	Route	Action	Side effect	Nursing Intervention

Diet Plan

24 hours nutritional requirements

Type of diet required (snacks, lunch, dinner)

Time	`Type	Quantity	Frequency	Remarks

List of Nursing Diagnosis/Problems/Need Identified According to Priority

1. --
2. --
3. --
4. --
5. --
6. --
7. --
8. --
9. --
10. --

Nursing Care Plan

Minimum of five problems should be addressed in your care plan

Nursing assessment (observation)	Nursing diagnosis	Objectives	Nursing intervention /action	Rationale	Evaluation
Subjective data What patient complains (symptoms) **Objective data** What nurse observes (signs)			Carrying planned nursing actions	Scientific principles	Problem resolved /result of intervention

Conclusion

Health education --

Nursing Case Study Format

Demographic data, nursing history, physical examination as per the format physical examination given in this text.

(Nursing assessment frequency and extent of the nursing assessment of any system function are based on several factors, including the severity of the patient's symptoms and presence of risk factors).

Includes above nursing care plan, and compares patient condition with theory knowledge of disease condition wherever applicable.

Diagnosis --

	Theory knowledge of disease condition of patient (as per text)	Present patient condition
Definition		
Related anatomy and physiology		
Etiology		
Risk factors		
Clinical manifestation		
Pathophysiology		
Assessment and diagnostic findings		
Medical management		
Nursing management		
Evaluation		
Health education		
Summary		
References		

Interactions with Special Clients

When interacting with an anxious client, recognize client's decreased ability to focus on and respond to multiple stimuli.

- Maintain quiet, calm environment
- Keep massage simple, concrete and brief
- Repeat messages often
- Minimize need for extensive decision making
- Monitor anxiety levels, using verbal and non-verbal cues when interacting with an angry client
- Use careful, unhurried, deliberate body movements
- Provide an open, non-threatening environment
- Maintain a non-threatening demeanor, using open body language soft voice tones and so forth.

When Interacting with a Client Exhibiting Denial

- Use direct question to determine the situation triggering use of coping mechanism

- Do not avoid the reality of the situation, but allow client to maintain denial defense, it often serves a protective function
- Recognize that denial may be the first of a series of crisis phase, to be followed by phases of increased tension, disorganization, attempts to recognize, attempts to escape the problem.

Blocks to Therapeutic Communication

- Giving advice
- Using responses that imply approval or disapproval
- Agreeing or disagreeing
- Not listening attentively
- Appearing distracted
- Imposing judgment
- Stereotyping
- Providing false assurance
- Excessive probing
- Questioning without basis
- Responding defensively.